YOUR CAREER AS A

DENTAL HYGIENIST

HEALTHCARE PROFESSIONAL

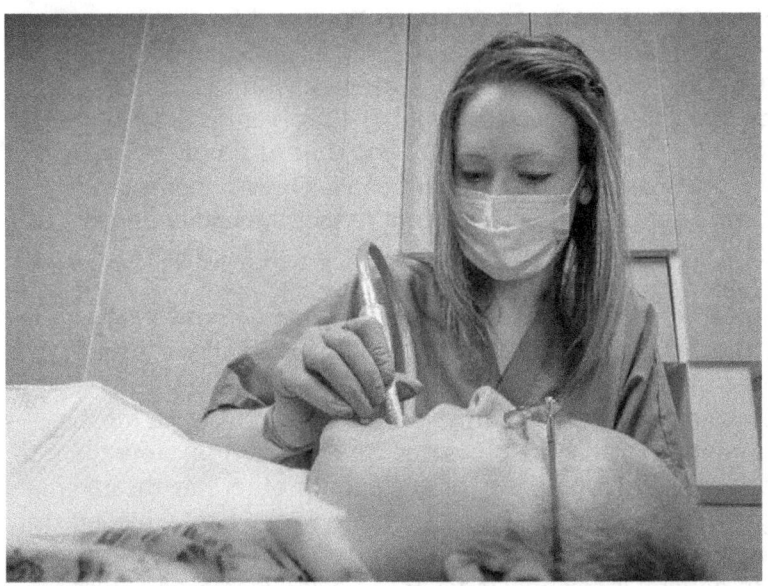

DENTAL HYGIENIST IS ONE OF THE most challenging healthcare careers. It is both physically and emotionally demanding and also requires a high level of intelligence. At the same time, it is a highly rewarding profession, providing the dental hygienist with opportunities to help many children and adults on the path to better health.

To excel as a dental hygienist you must have stamina, dexterity, and intense concentration. You must be a skilled visual observer and also a good listener, able to pay attention to detail and sort out the important data. In addition, you must be able to interact well with both colleagues and patients and, with the patients, have the ability to explain what you are doing when treating them and what they need to do to maintain their own dental well-being. This educational aspect of the work is viewed by many dental hygienists as the most important component of their work. In fact, dental hygienists are in some ways the most important health educators with whom many people ever come in contact.

Above all, you must have an empathetic nature, understanding that the patients you see are often in pain. You must be able to put them at ease, to the greatest degree possible under the circumstances, and proceed with your work with the utmost delicacy and care. For many patients, the problem is not pain as much as it is fear, not necessarily of you, but of simply being in a dentist's office and in the treatment chair. These patients require your compassion. Their fears may not reflect the reality of the experience, but they are nonetheless real for those patients.

This is a career that offers independence, even when working under the auspices of a dental practice. Hygienists work alone, usually in their own treatment rooms. While many states in the US still require that a hygienist work in a dentist's office, in recent years most states and many Canadian provinces have decided to allow them to work out of their own offices, or in clinics or other healthcare settings without the presence of a dentist. Many dental hygienists are extremely excited about these changes. They note that the public in general is strongly in favor of having increased access to healthcare professionals, especially those working with under-served populations. It is a promising development for these communities to have access to easy, convenient, affordable dental care. As these changes take place, the availability of dental hygiene in schools, hospitals, nursing homes, and programs such as Head Start, can lead to a fundamental change in the overall health of the nation, with the cost of dental care reduced because of the preventative work that is being done.

All of this makes it a great time to be joining the dental hygiene profession! It is possible that there will be a shortage as the demand for dental hygienists will be high in the coming years. Dental hygienists tend to make more than other healthcare professionals with similar levels of education and responsibilities.

Of course, there will be differences from state to state, and between urban and rural regions. Even with the demand, you may not find exactly the right job the first time you look, but with so much happening in the profession, it is a great time to be looking for that perfect fit.

THINGS TO DO NOW

THERE IS A STRONG POSSIBILITY THAT your interest in this profession came from your interaction with the dental hygienist who has taken care of your teeth. If that is the case, you should not hesitate to ask for advice and guidance about how to prepare for joining the profession. Hygienists can talk to you in detail about the work they do, the educational program they went through, and how they went about finding their first job. They can also offer advice about what steps you can take while still in high school to help you prepare for college.

Your dental hygienist can also provide you with a plan for taking care of your own dental health. In a sense, you will be providing a model for your future patients to follow. In addition, you can discover where the difficulties arise in sticking to a dental health regimen. This can be very helpful in preparing you to understand the challenges your patients will face in following through on the assignments you give to them and how to support them in sticking to their dental health efforts.

You should also contact your state and local dental hygienist associations. While you may not be able to become a member as yet, you can ask them to let you know about any relevant lectures or conferences in your area. You might be able to volunteer to help at events, which would be a great way to get your professional networking underway.

In your school you can begin preparing for this career by making sure you take classes in biology, chemistry, and mathematics. In addition, it will be useful to take classes in English to work on your communications skills, as so much of your work will involve educating your patients about dental health. Studying a foreign language can also be useful, as you may wind up serving one of the growing ethnic communities in the US. Another thing you can do in your school would be to work with your school nurse to establish a dental health club.

You should also consider using the physical education facilities of your school to begin an exercise program that focuses on stamina and flexibility. Being a dental hygienist does not usually require physical strength in terms of being able to lift heavy objects. It does mean that you will be standing for long periods, often in a bent over position. Playing sports is useful, too, as it is a way to develop your hand-eye coordination.

Learning to play a musical instrument is another way to prepare for a career as a dental hygienist. Playing a guitar or the piano, or just about any instrument helps to develop dexterity.

For information about accredited programs and educational requirements, it would be very useful to visit the website of the American Dental Hygienists' Association (ADHA). The State Board of Dental Examiners in each state can provide information on licensing requirements.

HISTORY OF DENTAL HYGIENIST AS A CAREER

THE DENTAL PROFESSION TRACES ITS roots back some 9,000 years to ancient India. Dentistry was practiced in ancient Egypt, in the classical period in Greece and Rome, through the Middle Ages and the Renaissance, and into the modern era. But it was only in the 1880s that dentists began providing preventive care for teeth and employing dental hygienists, who were first referred to as dental nurses, to be responsible for that care.

The title dental hygienist was created by Dr. Alfred C. Fones in 1906, when he trained his cousin Irene Newman to be his assistant, specifically charged with scaling and polishing teeth. Their teamwork proved popular with patients and the two opened a school in Connecticut to train dental hygienists. With several dozen students graduating, the state decided that there should be a licensing procedure to ensure that everyone working in this new profession was qualified to practice. The dental profession, concerned that hygienists might begin performing some of the tasks associated with dentistry, lobbied the Connecticut state government to put boundaries on the work that dental hygienists might do, so that by 1915, the state was both licensing and regulating dental hygienists. Dentists in other states viewed the Connecticut situation favorably and soon most states were adding licensing demands and regulatory rules for dental hygienists.

Dental hygienists began forming their own state associations, and soon joined together to create the national organization that still exists today, the American Dental Hygienists' Association (ADHA).

Regulation at the national level started in 1962 with the first national board exam for dental hygienists. The 1960s also saw the first men joining a profession that had previously been all women.

A key development for dental hygienists took place in the 1970s, when the first dental hygienist was appointed to a state board of dentistry, a great step forward in recognition and respect. Another big advance in this period, in terms of the right of women workers to be comfortable, was a change in the standard uniform worn by dental hygienists, allowing them to wear pants instead of dresses. Another development in this period was the decision by a majority of state regulatory boards to allow dental hygienists to administer local anesthesia.

The 1980s saw key changes in the interaction of dental hygienists with their patients in terms of safety. The Occupational Safety and Health Administration (OSHA) provided recommendations for infection control and also mandated changes in sterilization and personal protection equipment (PPE). Gloves, eyewear, and a mask were now required while providing dental treatment. Many of these developments were driven by the AIDS epidemic and heightened concerns that the disease could be spread through the interaction of dentists and dental hygienists, and their patients.

Over the past 30 years the development in the profession of dental hygienist has largely been along the lines of added responsibilities in the use of new, advanced equipment such as digital radiography for analyzing patient conditions. Another major advance has been the demand for esthetic services such as veneers and teeth whitening.

WHERE YOU WILL WORK

THE VAST MAJORITY OF REGISTERED dental hygienists in the US and Canada work in dental offices alongside dentists. In the US this is almost exclusively the case. The exceptions are in a handful of states, such as Maine, Minnesota, New Mexico, and Oregon that are experimenting with allowing dental hygienists to work in health clinics in rural areas, in nursing homes and long-term-care facilities, and in dental hygiene group practice clinics that do not include a dentist.

For dental hygienists who are inclined to pursue a more academic route in addition to or as an alternative to practicing their profession, opportunities exist in teaching. This avenue does require that the practitioner obtain a bachelor's and then a master's degree in dental hygiene.

Earning an advanced degree also opens the door to a career in research. This can take place in an academic setting or with one of the companies that provide products to the dental care industry, everything ranging from toothpaste, tooth brushes, and dental floss, up to more advanced electronic diagnostic equipment or even to the types of furniture that allow the most comfortable interaction of patient and hygienist.

In most instances, dental hygienists work in the clean, well lit, and comfortable environments that are found in the typical treatment room of a dental practice. For those who provide mobile services, this may not always be the case if, for example, they are visiting a home bound patient or working in a public health clinic where funding is limited.

In smaller dental practices, the hygienist may use the same treatment room where the dentist works. In larger practices, the hygienist space can be a room that is strictly for hygiene treatment and is not encumbered with the more extensive equipment used by a dentist.

THE WORK YOU WILL DO

MOST DENTAL HYGIENISTS WORK IN dentist practices typically serving one to two patients per hour. That is about the same pace for those who might work in a clinical setting, although hygienists who have their own practices may want to work at a slower pace.

Since each state has its own specific regulations regarding the range of services performed by dental hygienists, not everyone will experience the same routine. In some states, for instance, hygienists may put in place temporary fillings and apply periodontal dressings. The following is a general description of the activities most likely to be performed by all hygienists.

At the beginning of the day, the dental hygienist makes sure that everything that might be needed is readily available – products, equipment, and literature, as well as the specific information, charts, x-rays, and other data about the patients to be seen that day. The workspace must be clean and ready to be used.

When a patient arrives, the hygienist begins with a health assessment, updating the ongoing health history record and inquiring about any specific dental concerns. Some hygienists take the patient's blood pressure and pulse, just to get a sense of any peculiarities that might be occurring in the moment. They may also want to conduct a head and neck inspection, seeking out any sore spots that might be related to dental conditions, and also to be prepared for any discomfort the patient might be exposed to during the treatment.

At this time, the hygienist would also take any X-rays that might be needed to check for cavities and other signs of damage and decay not readily visible to the naked eye. Hygienists also use their own eyes to look for the more obvious signs of oral diseases such as gingivitis. An oral cancer exam or screening might be administered if there is any suggestion of its need, including a history of tobacco use by the patient.

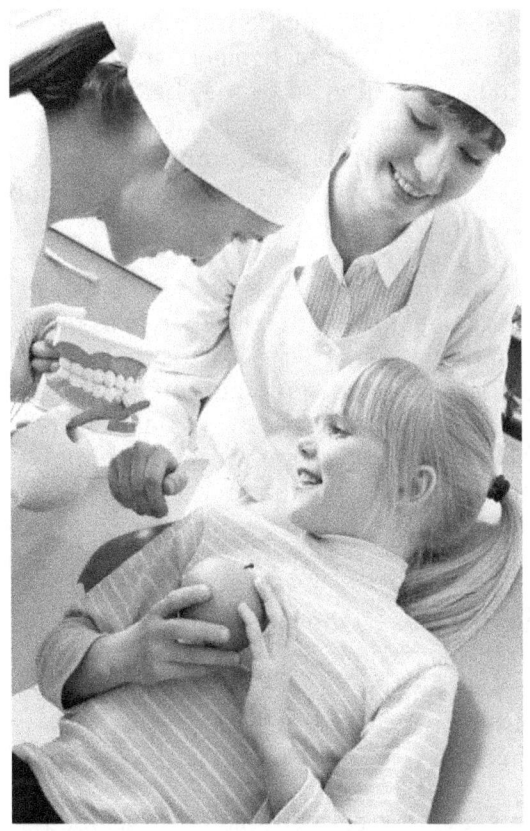

Once finished with the preliminary examination, the hygienist then begins instrumentation, searching for plaque and tartar with hand-held mouth mirrors, then using metal scalers and curettes (scalers with rounded ends for use under the gum line), to scrape away and remove deposits from surfaces and under the gum line. In the course of performing these tasks, dental hygienists wear safety glasses and surgical masks, as well as surgical-type gloves to protect themselves and patients from infectious diseases.

In some cases, the hygienist will use an ultrasonic scraper, an electronic device that uses vibrations to break up the plaque and tartar. This is a better method for patients who have very sensitive mouths and teeth, or who are extremely nervous and uncomfortable about having their teeth worked on.

To relieve the patient's anxiety, dental hygienists will typically accompany the instrumentation period with a steady stream of conversation, taking the opportunity to educate the patient about what they are doing and why they are doing it. It is also an occasion to provide an assessment of what they see in the patient's mouth, both good and bad, laying the groundwork for their recommendations regarding the regimen of dental care the patient should follow until the next cleaning.

If there is some infection or some damage inside the mouth that suggests that infection is possible, the dental hygienist may administer antibiotics or other medications. This may be done independently or under the direct supervision of the dentist with whom the hygienist is working. It is possible that some work will require the patient to have local anesthesia, and it would be the job of the hygienist to administer that.

Once the instrumentation work has been completed, the hygienist will usually polish or brush the patient's teeth, and then floss them. Polishing can be done by hand, but it is often a process that involves a tool that is essentially a very powerful automatic toothbrush. The hygienist may also work at removing stains, usually by employing an air-polishing device, which sprays a combination of air, water, and baking soda. It is possible that in this phase, the hygienist would apply sealants to give certain teeth better protection, and fluoride as an additional preventive measure.

There is usually an ongoing narrative by the hygienist while this work is taking place. When the cleaning is done, the hygienist continues the conversation with an emphasis on what the patient can do at home to contribute to dental health, including a review of brushing and flossing techniques.

If there are specific problems, then a treatment plan is developed between the hygienist and the patient. Dental hygienists, while not nutritionists, can also discuss their patients' eating habits and offer counseling on diet that shifts the patient's food intake away from any specific things that are bad for their teeth in general or for a specific problem with which the patient is dealing.

In some instances, it might be appropriate to make a cast of the patient's teeth to document an obvious surface or structural problem so that the dentist can study it and determine a course of action suited to the required treatment.

Many hygienists will escort the patient to the reception area to oversee making the next appointment. At this point, the dental hygienist wraps up the visit by performing documentation, entering clinical notes and processing office management paperwork for the patient's records. The hygienist then will clean the workspace, sterilizing instruments and making sure the area is prepared for the next appointment.

Unless hygienists have been able to plan out a schedule that has them in only one office every day, they may spend some time each day driving between offices. This is because so many dental hygienists work part time at a number of offices. Driving is also a part of the job for those hygienists who work outside of an office in a mobile unit that is outfitted as a treatment room on wheels. In addition, hygienists who do clinical work may find themselves driving long distances in rural areas to visit out-of-the-way patients for whom accessing a dental practice is extremely difficult.

Dental hygienists who go on to work in academia will have many of the same responsibilities of other teachers, preparing lessons and grading papers. They will also typically have some clinical responsibilities, guiding their students through hands-on training in dental hygiene practices.

Those dental hygienists who go to work for corporations may become involved in laboratory research, developing new products that could range from manual and electronic instruments, to polishing or brushing compounds. For those with a strong science interest this may be the ultimate path to follow. Alternatively, going to work for a company engaged in making the products and supplies used by hygienists could mean becoming involved in sales and marketing. Work of this nature typically involves travel and strong spoken and written communications skills.

DENTAL HYGIENISTS TALK ABOUT THEIR CAREERS

I Became Interested in Becoming a Dental Hygienist After a Visit to Get My Teeth Cleaned and Was Impressed by the Hygienist

"I was already thinking of a career in healthcare. It was dental hygienist or nursing, and I got accepted in dental hygiene first. I love being a dental hygienist because I get to help people every day become healthier, immediately. It's very rewarding seeing someone improve their health because of the education and therapy you deliver.

Dental hygienists are healthcare professionals who specialize in helping people with their oral health. I believe the most important part of my job is to help people understand how important it is to care for their teeth as part of staying healthy. I clean their teeth thoroughly so they have a base line to strive to achieve every day on their own.

I believe you have to be an empathic person who understands that you will be meeting people from all walks of life so you have to be able to read body language, understand cultural differences, and help them become comfortable in the dental hygiene chair. You will be dealing with a very intimate part of a person's body so sensitivity is important. You have to have good dexterity. You will be working by looking at the reflection in the mirror. You must be OK with blood and a person's reaction to pain. You need a really good sense of touch because you will be working in a very small space where you often can't see what you are doing.

It is a challenge to stay healthy over your career. You have to be willing to take care of your body because these workers typically have bad backs, wrists, and shoulders over time. It's also a challenge to put into practice everything you've learned, all of it. Most hygienists over time become time stressed by employers so they end up cutting corners, skipping the flossing or not doing a great job. Staying motivated under these conditions can be very hard."

I Had a Bad Dental Experience as a Child

"I decided to go to school for dental hygiene so I could help other people avoid what happened to me. I always knew I wanted to have a job that allowed me to help people in the community. I saw this as a good opportunity, and I love my career choice.

I provide oral healthcare screenings, prophylaxis, radiographs, fluoride treatments, sealants. I'm also responsible for charting, medical history intake, scheduling, sterilizing instruments and other jobs within the office. I do want to point out that the specific tasks can vary from office to office, and also by state, because there are different regulations in different places.

Wherever they work, a person interested in this career should be able to multi-task, like talking to patients while you are working in their mouth, have a passion for healthcare, master good time management, and be able to work under stress. This career is fast changing and requires a person to be flexible and able to go with the flow while maintaining a positive attitude and smiling face. Patients need to feel that they can trust you and that you can give them the best care.

I love helping people. I love working in public health and I work with many underprivileged patients. This is the greatest reward. The people in the community are so grateful for the help and services that are being provided to them, otherwise they would most likely go without care. I also feel that educating children on oral healthcare is very rewarding as well!

While helping people is amazing, it can also be very challenging and upsetting. The vulnerability in some patients that I see daily tugs at my heartstrings, and you have to deal with the fact that you did all you could and that you made a positive impact on their lives. Other challenges could be ethical. For example, you may not agree with the dentist's treatment plans or issues inside the office where you work. All I can say is do what you think is best and protect yourself. If you find yourself not fitting in somewhere, just keep looking. The right fit for you is out there.

Dental hygiene is changing, evolving, and about to make our profession much more important. With workforce models like Advanced Dental Hygiene Practitioner and Midlevel Provider happening in certain states, it is only a matter of time before it is the case nationwide. This will create more jobs, but more importantly it will help with access to care!"

I Became Interested in Becoming a Dental Hygienist While in High School

"I was very intimidated by the amount of science in the curriculum so initially I went to school for business administration. My desire to be a dental hygienist never went away, so I went back to school to pursue this career when I was in my 40s. It was not only the hardest thing I have done in my life, but the most rewarding!

I work with our patients to help them to achieve optimal oral health. A typical appointment starts with reviewing the patient's medical history, checking blood pressure, reviewing or taking radiographs, checking their periodontal status, performing an extraoral and intraoral exam, and an oral cancer exam. At this point you can make a dental hygiene diagnosis and know what procedures will come next, usually prophylaxis, scaling and root planing, and periodontal maintenance. At some point, the dentist will also do an exam determining a complete diagnosis.

A big part of this entire process is educating the patient regarding proper brushing, flossing and oral healthcare. It is frustrating that patients don't floss on a regular basis. They listen and appear to understand how important it is, but cannot find the time, even though it only takes about a minute to floss daily!

Working with patients, teaching them that oral health is related to overall health is the best part of my job. For anyone in this career, it's really important to enjoy working with people. You also need to love science, and have the determination to understand it!"

I Got to Talking With My Family Dentist During One of My Routine Visits and I Was Offered a Part-Time Position for After School and on Saturdays

"In my practice today, I spend a lot of time in the education of my patients on everything from tobacco cessation, nutritional counseling, wear and tear to the teeth and how that relates to airway issues, the oral systemic link relative to heart disease, diabetes, low birth rate babies, radiographs, prophylaxis, local anesthesia, fluoride, soft tissue management and periodontal scaling, and sealants.

I am passionate about passing on as much of my knowledge as possible to my patients and seeing that knowledge empowers them. It can be tough finding ways to help patients value the information we share with them, so that they take responsibility for their health.

I also love learning from other hygienists through national and local continuing education meetings. Joining ADHA has been one of the best long-term investments I have made. Through my membership, I have gained more opportunities and top notch mentoring, not to mention discounts on numerous things.

So much is happening it is hard to keep up, but you have to. You must have the desire to continually learn and stay abreast of the latest research and advances in your profession. It is an exciting time to be a dental hygienist as we try to expand what we do and where we are able to do it. One of the biggest obstacles is to have legislation and regulations keep up with the demands of the times for Access to Care issues. We need to get to the point where we can legally practice what we have been trained with our education to do.

I recommend that young people take full advantage of the education and training they receive at school, yet remember that every day is a learning experience! Always be familiar with advances in the field, the newest technology and products. As a past president of my state association, I can tell you that a great way to do this is by being actively involved in your state's professional association and the national association, the American Dental Hygienists' Association."

I Was Always Interested in Teeth

"As a Registered Dental Hygienist I'm able to perform cleanings, which can consist of regular routine cleanings or deep cleanings/scaling, take x-rays, provide oral hygiene education, give local anesthesia, fluoride treatments, dental screening which includes oral cancer screenings, checking for possible cavities, or signs of other diseases/conditions etc.

Most hygienists I know are personable, and have a passion for dental hygiene and helping others improve their quality of life. When working with children, I am able to ease a child's fear of the unknown, when it is the first visit to the office. To see a smile on a child's face after their appointment is heaven.

It's also great to work with adults and be able to teach them something new that they've never heard before. Then on the next visit they remember what we talked about.

Skills should include being able to multi-task, having good dexterity, and being able to work with people from all walks of life. You need to be open enough to identify the obstacles you face and flexible enough to adjust so that these challenges and difficulties can no longer hold you back."

I Filled Out an Occupational Interest Survey While in High School and Was Given the Opportunity to Join an Explorer Scout Troop That Was Dental Based

"I originally did not think I was going to go to college, so I started looking at vocational education through my high school. With the Scout group I was given the opportunity to observe in a dental office and learn about the different positions available in the dental team. I found myself being drawn to the dental hygienist's room and decided that's what I wanted to do.

I now work in a community health center, so I specifically work with clients that have diabetes, heart disease, and HIV. I am the preventive specialist in the center. I educate my patients on gum disease, and how to treat and prevent disease and decay. I educate on the body-mouth connection and how overall health and dental health are related. In addition, I perform prophy (prophylactic teeth cleaning), root planing and scaling procedures, sealants, fluoride treatments, and nutritional counseling for preventing decay.

I get a lot of happiness out of knowing that I am helping

patients improve and maintain not only their oral health, but also their overall health. I also love when patients get finished with their appointment and they smile so big because their teeth feel so good! It makes me wish I had more time to spend with my patients, to make sure everything is perfect.

I also wish there were more opportunities for dental hygienists to work in clinics. There are few full-time positions, and a lot of my friends have to work several part-time jobs or fill in at temporary positions. I feel the future is bright though, and that there will be greater opportunity to reach clients that don't currently receive dental hygiene care, including nursing home care, work in schools, head start programs, WIC centers and beyond.

I feel that there are opportunities in the future we may not have even considered, as dental hygiene duties expand and the demand for quality dental hygiene care increases. One thing I do think will happen is there will be more opportunities to work closely with other medical professionals.

I would encourage all dental hygiene students to pursue further education beyond their entry-level dental hygiene degree. There are opportunities outside of clinical dental hygiene that include teaching, sales, presenting continuing education seminars, research, administration and beyond."

PERSONAL QUALIFICATIONS

DENTAL HYGIENISTS NEED TO BE excellent communicators. A big part of their job is educating their patients, children, as well as adults, about home care and maintenance of their teeth, conveying information in terms that the patients can understand and be willing to follow. Their communications skills also come into play as they work on their patients explaining what they are doing while they are doing it, in ways that are comforting and able to ease the patient's concerns and fears.

Dental hygienists must also be skilled listeners, able to hear and react immediately when a patient indicates discomfort. In order to communicate in this manner dental hygienists should have a high level of compassion for their patients. They are dealing with people who may be afraid and could also be in severe pain.

Being able to reassure patients that the procedures are going well should be born out of the dental hygienist's self-confidence. Because of the importance of the healthcare being provided, the intimacy of the experience, and the precision required, the hygienist must continually reassure the patient.

This is also a profession that demands a high level of organizational skills. Dental hygienists handle a large assortment of tools and, since they tend to work individually without any assistance, they need to keep their equipment in good order and ready for use. Related to this skill is the requirement that guidelines set out by the state governing boards and professional associations are strictly adhered to.

Dental hygienists make a point of the physical demands of their work, as well as the intellectual, social, and emotional aspects. They must be good at working with their hands, with a considerable amount of dexterity, and good hand and eye coordination. Dental hygienists generally work in tight quarters on a small part of the body, using very precise tools and instruments. Physical stamina and flexibility are a must, given that you will spend a large percent of your time bending over patients as you work on their mouths.

Other important personal qualifications include a positive disposition that lends itself to interacting on good terms with a small group of coworkers in a relatively confined environment, given that dental practices are rarely in large office suites.

A love of science is also an important trait. Dental hygienists need to understand detailed information about the biology and chemistry of the human body and also know the science behind the materials they use.

ATTRACTIVE FEATURES

DENTAL HYGIENISTS GET A HIGH LEVEL of satisfaction from helping their patients live healthier lives. The work of cleaning teeth provides immediate gratification, while being able to teach people good practices to use on their own to improve their oral health adds to the satisfaction. This holds true for adult patients, and it can be even truer when helping children to learn good dental practices.

Hand in hand with their core task of maintaining the oral health of patients, is the challenge of helping them, especially children, to overcome their fear of going to the dentist. By providing a comforting presence, dental hygienists play a key role in making what is often one of the most uncomfortable situations that people find themselves in, something that feels worthwhile. Having the opportunity to establish trusting relationships with patients, young and old alike, is one of the most appealing aspects of this work.

In general, dental hygienists are respected for the work they do. Patients recognize how hard working, diligent, and skilled their individual hygienists are, and this translates to a broader, overall positive feeling about the profession.

This is also a career that offers an interesting blend of routine and variety, satisfying the needs of both types of personalities. The tasks performed are generally routine, but each individual patient offers unique challenges due to age, physique, emotional and intellectual status, overall health, and dental health.

Added to this is the change taking place in the profession in terms of more and more states allowing hygienists to work on their own without the supervision of a dentist and in locations where they have not worked previously, such as health clinics, mobile facilities, and even out of their own dedicated offices.

The profession of dental hygienist also offers a substantial degree of security, as good practitioners are always in demand. A rapid rate of growth is predicted for the profession over the coming years, well above the average for all occupations.

UNATTRACTIVE ASPECTS

BEING A DENTAL HYGIENIST IS BOTH A physically and mentally challenging career. The work requires a very high degree of concentration, a steady hand, and a willingness to engage emotionally with your patients. At the end of the day you can find yourself drained. This is no doubt a contributing factor to why so many dental hygienists only work part time, and why some struggle to maintain their motivation.

There is often stress related to the workplace that has nothing to do with the work itself. It can result from the dynamics of working in an environment where everyone is under pressure to perform very exacting kinds of tasks, while maintaining a very upbeat and calm facade for the patients. This kind of stress is one of the motivating factors in the desire of some dental hygienists to start their own practices. Of course, taking the step to become financially independent rather than an employee in someone else's practice can create even greater stress. You discover that you must deal with financing your business, making insurance payments, publicizing and marketing, and attracting a group of regular patients. As dental hygienists are permitted to become independent in the coming years they will face even greater challenges.

Dental hygienists are happiest when their patients show up with teeth that have been cared for at home. The worst part of the job is seeing returning patients that have not paid any attention to the preventive care instructions they were given at their previous appointments. This situation, while very common, is nevertheless extremely frustrating.

EDUCATION AND TRAINING

DENTAL HYGIENISTS TYPICALLY EARN an associate degree or a certificate in order to qualify for professional licensing. Some prefer to go on for bachelor's and master's degrees as well. The end goal of the educational process is to be prepared to take a state licensing exam. Every state requires dental hygienists to be licensed. Requirements vary by state, but in most states, a degree from an accredited dental hygiene program and passing grades on written and practical examinations are required for licensure. For specific application requirements, contact your state's medical or health board.

According to the American Dental Hygienists Association, there are more than 330 accredited dental hygiene programs in the US, including about 200 that offer an associate degree. In Canada, there are four universities and 33 colleges offering degrees to dental hygienists.

Programs typically cover both the theoretical foundation supporting the practice of dental hygiene, along with hands-on work in classrooms and clinical settings. By the time they graduate, students are expected to be able to perform every task required of a dental hygienist. Upon completion of the required number of program credits, a student can apply to take the National Board Dental Hygiene Examination and, assuming successful completion of that exam, take the state licensing exam.

Students in a dental hygiene program are taught such practical skills as how to:

- Document medical and dental histories

- Perform head and neck cancer screenings

- Take X-rays

- Place temporary fillings

- Finish and polish amalgam restorations

- Scale and polish teeth

- Apply preventative agents

Students also get instruction in how to be educators themselves, teaching their patients about oral health and prevention.

Student members of the ADHA are assigned a student advisor who can be of great assistance as you move through your college program.

Associate Degree and Certificate Programs

There is little difference between a dental hygiene associate degree and certificate programs. Both prepare the student to take the national licensing exam, a local clinical exam, and the state licensing exam. Among the specific courses found in both types of programs are:

- Anatomy & Physiology for Hygienists

- Anesthesia

- Basic Psychology

- Communications

- Community Dentistry

- Dental Biochemistry

- Dental Emergencies & Pathology

- Dental Hygiene Clinic Operations

- Dental Materials

- Dental Practice: Ethics and Management

- General Pathology

- Head/Neck Anatomy & Embryology

- Health Promotion

- Introduction to Dental Hygiene

- Nutrition & Dental Health

- Oral Histology & Embryology

- Oral Pathology

- Periodontology

- Pharmacology and Pain Management

- Preventive Dental Practices

- Principles of Dental Hygiene

- Principles of Microbiology

- Public Health Dentistry

- Radiology

- Special Needs Dentistry

Bachelor's and Master's Degrees

Graduates holding associate degrees or certificates in dental hygiene can apply for a degree completion program that will lead to a bachelor's degree. Earning a degree gives dental hygienists additional career opportunities in business, sales, education, research, and public health. Many of the completion programs are offered on a part-time basis as well as full time, and at some schools classes are often scheduled for evenings and weekends. It is assumed the student will continue to be a working dental hygienist while pursuing a degree, and some programs will develop a schedule that suits the individual's work schedule.

Course work towards a bachelor's degree requires taking classes in such non-dental hygiene areas as mathematics, writing, humanities, social sciences, literature, history, and international studies. The additional dental courses can include:

- Allied Health Education

- Health Management Practicum

- Nursing Research

- Research Methods

- Social Research Methods

The master's degree adds credibility to one's career and is a great aid in landing any position you choose to pursue. For many dental hygienists the purpose of taking an advanced degree is a matter of personal satisfaction and a sign of commitment to the profession. Some dental hygienists pursue higher degrees in public health, seeking to combine their special area of concern, dental hygiene, with the larger issue of public health.

Licensing

All states require dental hygienists to be licensed. The requirements can vary from state-to-state, so it is best to contact your state's Board of Dental Examiners, which can provide information on licensing requirements. The job of the board is to ensure that all practicing dental professionals have an appropriate level of education and training, and that high professional standards are maintained.

Each individual applicant's education and training are verified by board staff. It is not uncommon for a board to conduct a background check to ensure that applicants who hold a license in another state are of good professional reputation and standing.

Boards typically require applicants to pass comprehensive written and clinical examinations. The written exam used for dental hygienists is the National Board Dental Hygiene Examination created and administered by the Joint Commission on National Dental Examinations. The 15-member Commission includes representatives from dental schools, dental practice, state dental examining boards, dental hygiene, dental students, and the public. The ADHA offers a live, online National Dental Hygiene Board Review course to help graduates prepare to take the licensure exam.

It is also fairly common for states to require that dental hygienists renew their licenses periodically, usually about every two years. Part of the renewal process is to demonstrate that the licensee has obtained the number of continuing education credits required by the board and that there have been no instances of unsafe or questionable practice or conduct reported on the applicant.

Education Costs

A dental hygiene program can be expensive, with some 20-month associate degree programs running in the $40,000 range. Therefore, choosing to pursue this career does require a significant financial commitment.

There are loans and scholarships available. For example, the American Dental Hygienists Association Institute for Oral Health (IOH) was created to provide educational scholarships and fellowships to dental hygienists throughout the country.

EARNINGS

THE MEDIAN ANNUAL SALARY FOR dental hygienists is about $75,000, and it has been rising. The top 10 percent of dental hygienists earn about $100,000. The bottom 10 percent earn about $50,000.

As you might expect, salaries are higher in urban centers where the cost of living is higher. California is notable for having salaries above the rest of the nation. The top-paid hygienists work in dental offices, but ambulatory healthcare services, where there are an increasing number of jobs available, also offer substantial salaries.

More than half of dental hygienists work part time, an ongoing situation for the profession. This is a bit misleading in that many hygienists work for two or more practices, scheduling a few hours at each one during a typical workweek. Even when working for multiple employers, dental hygienists are often less than fully employed. This presents a difficulty for those who are part-timers in that benefits such as paid vacation, sick leave, and contributions to their retirement fund are typically available only to full-time workers.

EMPLOYMENT OUTLOOK

EMPLOYMENT OF DENTAL HYGIENISTS IN the US is projected to grow over 30 percent within the coming decade. This is a much higher rate than the average for all occupations. Growth will be spurred by an increasing awareness within the healthcare community and among the general population, that dental health is a crucial component of overall health and well-being.

Another factor includes an anticipated expansion of insurance coverage for dental care that will encourage greater numbers of people to seek these services, and especially preventive treatment, the specialty of the hygienist. This is coupled with an expanding population of people, especially seniors, who have teeth that need care. This is in contrast to previous generations where it was more common for people to have lost their teeth in their senior years.

Also contributing to the need for more hygienists will be the ongoing change in state regulations that will permit hygienists to work outside of dentist offices and without dentist supervision, either in their own dental hygiene practices, or in a wide variety of public and private healthcare facilities.

For some hygienists, there can be additional employment opportunities. If they are willing to stay up to date on new techniques and procedures there should be teaching opportunities as the demand for new hygienists grows. Academia also presents opportunities for working in research for the development of new products and practices.

There will be opportunities for hygienists to work for private corporations that are engaged in creating, manufacturing, and marketing dental materials and equipment.

GETTING STARTED

FINDING YOUR FIRST JOB COULD HAVE much to do with where you are located and if you are willing to relocate. In either case, your opportunities will largely rest upon your own efforts, first to excel in your studies, and then to move as quickly as possible to obtain the certifications required to practice in your state. Next, you will need to use the available resources of local, state, and national associations to identify opportunities, and to network as much as possible at association meetings and conventions, as well as through online social media. Membership in associations can be invaluable not just for networking but for keeping up with technical and professional developments in dental hygiene. You can become a student member of the ADHA if you are enrolled in an accredited dental hygiene program.

The job-hunting effort will require research on the numbers and density of dentist offices and hygienists in an area. If your state has decided to allow dental hygienists to work independently in settings other than a dentist's office, you can expand your search to include public and private health clinics, senior citizen facilities, schools, and other venues in which the services of a dental hygienist are likely to be desired.

Since this is a new opportunity in most areas in the US, these venues may not have a program set up for a dental hygienist. There may be opportunities to help develop programs from the ground up for the right creative go-getter.

You may want to become involved in community service activities as another networking venue and even go so far as to visit individual practices and make yourself known to the people working there. Do not hesitate to ask for advice from people with more experience, whether you are seeking information on opportunities in an area or just to have someone review your résumé.

Veteran dental hygienists advise newcomers to stay open to new experiences and not get stuck in expectations about what that first job will be like. They remind job hunters to have patience in looking for a job, of if they have accepted a first job that is not their ideal. They say do not get discouraged, keep searching, because the right job and the right fit are out there for you.

RESOURCES FOR STUDENTS

■ **American Academy of Periodontology**
www.perio.org

■ **American Dental Association**
www.ada.org/en

■ **American Dental Hygienists Association**
www.adha.org

■ **Canadian Dental Association**
www.cda-adc.ca/en

■ **Canadian Dental Hygienists Association**
www.cdha.ca

■ **International Federation of Dental Hygienists**
www.ifdh.org

■ **National Dental Hygienists Association**
www.ndhaonline.org

PUBLICATIONS

■ **ADA News**
www.ada.org/en/publications/ada-news

■ **Access Magazine**
www.adha.org/access-magazine

■ **Canadian Journal of Dental Hygiene**
www.cdha.ca

■ **CDC Essentials**
www.cda-adc.ca/en/services/essentials

■ **Dental Economics**
www.dentaleconomics.com/index.html

■ **Dental Product Guide**
www.ada.org/en/publications/ada-dental-product-guide

■ **Dentistry iQ**
www.dentistryiq.com/index.html

■ **Journal of Periodontology**
www.perio.org/journal.html

■ **Journal of the American Dental Association**
http://www.ada.org/en/publications/jada

■ **Journal of Dental Hygiene**
www.adha.org/jdh

■ **Perio-Implant Advisory**
www.perioimplantadvisory.com/index.html

■ **Professional Product Review**
www.ada.org/en/publications/ada-professional-product
-review-ppr/

■ **RDH**
www.rdhmag.com/index.html

www.ingramcontent.com/pod-product-compliance
Lightning Source LLC
Chambersburg PA
CBHW070429190526
45169CB00003B/1469